IBS Diet
Irritable Bowel Syndrome

The Ultimate Guide for
Lasting Control

Low Carb Way of Healthy Life
with IBS Diet

WaraWaran Roongruangsri

Pawana Publishing
Good Health Content

IBS Diet (Irritable Bowel Syndrome)

Without health, life is not life; it is only a state of languor and suffering.
- Francois Rabelais

First Publish in 2015 by Pawana Publishing
Copyright © 2015 WaraWaran Roongruangsri
Pawana © is a registered trademark of Pawana Publishing.
Cover and interior design by Pawana Publishing
Interior photos © Pawana Publishing
Author photo by Pawana Publishing

ISBN-13: 978-1517472962
ISBN-10: 1517472962

This document is geared towards providing exact and reliable information in regards to the topic and issue covered. The publication is sold with the idea that the publisher is not required to render accounting, officially permitted, or otherwise, qualified services. If advice is necessary, legal or professional, a practiced individual in the profession should be ordered.

- From a Declaration of Principles which was accepted and approved equally by a Committee of the American Bar Association and a Committee of Publishers and Associations.

In no way is it legal to reproduce, duplicate, or transmit any part of this document in either electronic means or in printed format. Recording of this publication is strictly

Author's Note

Irritable Bowel Syndrome, which is other ways called IBS, is a condition caused by the dysfunction of bowel. If you are diagnosed with IBS, you need to know how to get relief from the symptoms you suffer.

You may feel unhappy thinking that you are the only one who gets irritated after eating certain food items like fruits, vegetables, beans, yogurt etc. Well, you are not the only one suffering from it. It is estimated that IBS affects 15% of teens and adults.

The happy news is you can be perfectly alright, if you are ready to follow a new kind of diet for few weeks. In older days, high-fiber diet was suggested for IBS.

You can learn here about the foods that worsen the symptoms of IBS for free. In every issue of 'IBS Diet', you get to learn valuable information on diets to follow if you are suffering from IBS.

Here, in IBS Diet book, you will know more about

- What is Irritable Bowel Syndrome?
- Stress and IBS
- IBS and your Diet
- IBS and Elimination Diets
- Eat to beat IBS with these tips
- The Best IBS Diet Suggestions for all
- Herbal Therapy for IBS
- Probiotics for IBS
- Prevention

In this issue, you will get more knowledge on IBS, and also on tips to control symptoms of IBS. Moreover, you will read some helpful information on diets to follow ad also about certain food items, like herbs and probiotics, that will help you to enjoy your favorite foods again.

Furthermore, you will learn effective ways to prevent IBS. This also includes answers to few of best reader questions. In fact, the IBS diet book is an ultimate guide that answers the important question: What you can do and what foods you can eat when you suffer from IBS?

Thanks for downloading this book. I hope you enjoy reading it!

WaraWaran Roongruangsri

IBS Diet (Irritable Bowel Syndrome)

CONTENTS

"Tell me what you eat, and I will tell you who you are."

- Brillat-Savarin

.

CHAPTER 1

WHAT IS IRRITABLE BOWEL SYNDROME?

Irritable Bowel Syndrome is a condition that no one really wants to talk about and therefore many people lack information on it. It is a common disease that 50% of the people, who visit gastroenterologist, suffer from it.

If you suffer from IBS, you might know it causes great deal of pain and discomfort. You can live a normal and healthy life with IBS, provided you are better informed about the condition and its preventive measures. We aim to provide you valuable information regarding IBS, so that you can lead a healthy life. The first step is to understand what exactly irritable bowel syndrome is.
What is IBS?

IBS occurs due to the disorder in the function of your bowel. Due to this, the patient experiences abdominal pain, in addition to changes in normal bowel habits. The condition is also called spastic colon.

Symptoms of IBS

There are many symptoms that may lead to diagnosis of IBS. It varies in each individual. However, when you are more informed, it will be helpful for your doctor as well.

The most frequent symptoms of IBS includes
- Pain in the lower abdomen
- Bloating
- Pain that is relieved by defecation

Diarrhea and constipation may also occur and it may move from one extent to another in certain patients. A change in stool may also be a symptom of IBS. Other severe conditions include chronic fatigue syndrome, stress, chronic pelvic pain and fibromyalgia. Moreover, certain other health conditions like menstruation worsen the symptoms of IBS.

There are studies that show the link between IBS and mental condition. It also shows that IBS have both neurological and psychological components.
What to do if you have IBS?

If you think you have the symptoms of IBS, you need to get it diagnosed and confirmed by your doctor. Your doctor will likely track your bowel movements over a period of time and also monitor other conditions. The doctor may also look to certain points like:

1. Are you relieved from the pain after defecation?
2. When you feel this way, is there a change in the frequency of your stool?
3. When you are experiencing this pain, is there a change in the form or the way that your stool looks?

They will determine the variations and then likely reach a decision. Check out the following conditions.

- If you have more than three bowel movements per day or you have less than three movements per week, then it is considered abnormal.
- If you have hard or lumpy stool or you have a very loose and watery stool
- If you are straining, or you have an urgent need to go or you feel like you can not completely finish, it is abnormal.
- If there is any sign of mucus, it is abnormal.
- Also the feeling of pain in the abdomen or the feeling of being bloated is considered abnormal.

Doctor may request a blood check up, before reaching a final conclusion. With the help of a final thorough examination to rule out the possibility of any other disease, the doctor would likely confirm IBS.

IBS Diet (Irritable Bowel Syndrome)

CHAPTER 2

STRESS AND IBS

Stress is a factor that causes and worsens many health conditions including IBS. Your doctor may talk about the role of stress in your condition.

It has to be noted first and foremost that stress by itself does not cause IBS. Stress generates after a troubled lifestyle. The health and capacity to withstand the disease often gets worsened by high stress.

We cannot determine the exact cause of IBS. In fact, we can treat and control the symptoms of IBS. However, we can draw the conclusion that stress is a factor that worsens the symptoms of IBS.

How stress hurts?

Obviously, stress worsens the symptoms of IBS. When a healthy person stays in an ideal situation, stress is automatically controlled by body. The body is equipped with a pain inhibition system that becomes active when it suffers pain. In the case of patients with IBS, the right pain inhibition system does not get active due to stress, and pain will worsen.

Consider this example. If you had a long and stressful day, you will need a good meal and sleep by the end of the day. If you are under prolonged stress, you cannot get to relax easily.

Instead, you may eat a meal. If you are eating under stressful event or not, you will get an awful abdominal pain that is associated with IBS. For a person with IBS, this does not seem to be normal. The body does not turn off the pain function and as a result you will feel more pain during or after stress.

CHAPTER 3

IBS AND YOUR DIET

It is a common notion that IBS is caused due to lack of healthy diet. But the fact is, like stress, diet does not create the condition of IBS. But definitely, your diet will aggravate IBS.

For people with IBS, body will react intensively to certain food items. The body experiences increased level of intestinal muscle reaction and sensitivity. That makes clear that the food you take may worsen the symptoms of IBS. It is difficult to find the single element that causes irritation, but tension occurs as a general over reaction to food.

Food intake and IBS

The good thing is that you can control what you eat and thus lessen the worries caused by IBS. Certain items like fried food items, alcohol, caffeine and fatty foods commonly creates tension for IBS patients. It is also advisable not to consume too much food in one sitting.

Some specific types of sugar can create diarrhea and abdominal cramping in IBS patients. An example for it is sorbitol which is a sweetener in foods like gum sugar, candy sugar etc. Consuming these types of sugars will lead to the inability of bowel in absorption, which in turn will cause diarrhea.

Foods like beans, legumes, cauliflowers, lentils, Brussels sprouts, onions, bagels, cabbage and broccoli can intensify the gas symptoms of IBS. It is good to avoid all these foods as it may create bloating and increased gas.

However, foods affect each other in a different way. Some foods that cause irritation for you may function fine in another patient. It is very essential that you try to understand the foods that cause tension for you and try to avoid it.

Track your diet

Tracking your diet is the first step to take while you have to manage with IBS. You might know the food you take, but it is less likely that you realize the correlation between diet and IBS symptoms. The goal is to get to know the food that worsens the IBS systems.

You can take two to three week's time to track your diet. Note down each and every single food you took during the time. And you need to monitor how you feel before and after taking the food and know if you experience the symptoms of IBS.

CHAPTER 4

IBS AND ELIMINATION DIETS

Diet control for IBS

Once you monitor your food intakes and irritation occurrences, you can find the food that causes or worsens the IBS symptoms. Those food items should strictly be removed from the diet. It is very hard to exactly find out the particular element in your food that creates irritation.

Well, we suggest you to track your intake of food and symptoms you face with the help of a chart.

You may be concerned about the thought that you will lose the quality of life by avoiding certain foods. You need not worry on this as it is important to reduce the symptoms of IBS. Such food items that need to be eliminated are called Elimination diets. However, the removal of essential nutrients from food may put your health at risk. Some people may suffer anemia, osteoporosis, and even suffer vitamin and mineral deficiencies.

We recommend you to take advice from doctor regarding elimination diet and your IBS situation.

There are chances that your doctor may further ask you to do couple of tests for proper diagnosis. It may be allergy tests or internal endoscope or even lactose breathing test. The doctor will make sure that you do not suffer from any other disease as your IBS symptoms may become worse in such conditions. Here is a list of health conditions that worsens the symptoms of IBS:

- Gastro esophageal reflux which is caused by chronic reflux of gases in esophagus.
- Celiac Disease or gluten enteropathy, a condition in which there is a reaction between gluten and intestinal muscle linings.
- Lactose intolerance is caused when body loses its ability to digest milk.
- The immune system may respond to the food you eat and causes food allergies.
- Eosinophilic Gastroenteritis is yet another illness in which white blood cells enter GI tract. It is a rare condition caused as a reaction to the food intake.

Further Monitoring of Elimination Diet

It is very essential to be aware of the food you consume. The quantity of the food is important as well. Many individuals with IBS have realized that consumption of too much of food at one sitting had triggered the symptoms they suffer.

We often consume too much of food in one sitting, which is not recommended for good health. It causes digestive problems and also results in over weight of the body.
You must have read the example of an individual who eats

a full meal and getting IBS symptoms in the beginning of this book. The reaction happens due to the hyper sensitivity of body, which is caused by IBS. The body loses its ability to react to the pain and the person suffers extreme pain, just because of over eating.

Well, you may be doubtful about the right quantity of food intake which would be helpful in fighting against the symptoms of IBS. We suggest you to check the correct portion of food that you take each time.

Packaging labels may help in finding out the correct portion. While you take a package of 4 servings, you can divide it in four and pick up one for you. You will able to understand the portion of food you take in that way.

Advisable quantity of food

We have few suggestions for food items that you take normally on terms of quantity.
Fruit: Consider the size of a baseball.1 cup of fruit will be of similar size.

Salad: Same as fruits, 1 cup of salad will also be in the size of a baseball.

Bread: In case of bread, a serving means one slice.

Potato, rice, pasta: In all of this, one serving means half a cup, and will look similar to half the size of baseball.

Pancake: A pancake stands for a serving. Take it as the size of a compact disc.

Meats: For any kind of meats, 3 ounces would be enough for a serving. Meats may be of fish, poultry, beef, pork etc. Let us say it will be in the size of a deck of playing cards.

Fish: Be it grilled or baked fish, a serving will be around 3 ounces and as the size of a check that fits into a checkbook.

Ice cream: Imagine half the size of a baseball and it forms a serving of ice-cream.

Milk: 1 cup is enough for a serving.

Cheese: In case of cheese, one and half ounce means one serving.

Oils used for cooking or greens: For any oil that you use, 1teaspoon is enough for one serving.
After going through the quantity of food, you may realize how much more you eat each time. You might be over eating these food stuffs every time and getting irritation. You can control the symptoms of IBS, if you follow a diet with right quantity of food.

That's not enough!

You might feel the prescribed quantity of food might not be sufficient for the body. There are few factors that play a role in how much you eat.

- Woman need to eat less compared to man.
- If you are a person who is involved in higher level of physical activity for more than half an hour a day, you have to eat more to compensate.
- During young age, you have to consume more food, as it is essential for proper growth.
- If you are an elderly person, your food intake should be proportional to the amount of physical activity you do each day.

We recommend you to take advice from your family

doctor about the proper diet suitable for you as well as the quantity of food your body needs. If you want an average scale of quantity of food for a physically active man and woman, it will come around 2200 and 1800 calories a day respectively.

IBS Diet (Irritable Bowel Syndrome)

CHAPTER 5

EAT TO BEAT IBS WITH THESE TIPS

Tips for Eating Less

It may be difficult for you to limit the food intake and enter into new diet suddenly. We offer you few suggestions which would help you to get into a proper diet. Go through the following suggestions and try to implement in your life.

1. You should be aware of the quantity of food you take each time.
2. Take a plate of smaller size so that you will eat lesser quantity of food.
3. You should not finish off your food in haste, but learn to enjoy each bite.
4. Control your temptation to eat the leftover food by keeping limited quantity of food on table.
5. Avoid snacking in between meals and be aware of what you eat.

These tips help you to reduce the amount of food intake, and further you can monitor and control the food that worsens the symptoms of IBS.

Over limitation of food

You might know that it will be risky to over limit the food intake when it comes to IBS dietary restrictions. There is no need to get into that extent in food control. When you over limit yourself to such a degree, you are putting your health at risk. Moreover, diets plans that are too strict is much harder to follow and also you will not be able to stay longer on it. Furthermore, some of these diets may require a replacement among food groups. The diet should be in such a way that the nutrition intake is not affected.

A well-balanced diet is part of a healthy lifestyle. So you need to carefully avoid or limit the foods that worsen the IBS symptoms from your diet.

Often, IBS patients are asked to maintain strict diet. It is not advisable to follow it, unless your doctor recommends it for limiting your severe IBS conditions.

CHAPTER 6

THE BEST IBS DIET SUGGESTIONS FOR ALL

The diet restriction may differ from person to person. However, there are few suggestions from which everyone can benefit. Consider the following tips:

- Make sure you drink 8 glasses of water a day.
- Include foods that contain fiber in your diet.
- Keep alcohol and caffeine consumption low.
- Eat six meals of smaller quantities and avoid snacks in between meals.
- Limit foods that contain sorbitol and fructose in your diet.
- High fatty foods and fried foods should be avoided as much as possible.

Following these tricks will help you to improve diet, and overall health, and most importantly, reduces the symptoms of IBS. However, we recommend you to get proper advice from your doctor on maintaining healthy diet.

Fiber intake is important

Fiber is an important component of good diet. Too much of fiber intake may result in diarrhea whereas low intake will lead to constipation. It makes clear that you should be careful in the intake of fiber foods.

You can start with consuming variety of different types of fiber. The best source of fiber is fruits, whole grains vegetables etc and it is always better to get the fiber needed for your body from natural resources.

Your body needs fiber for several reasons. For example, fiber produces a gas which is necessary to stimulate your colon muscles as well as to soften your stool. In individuals with IBS, deficiency of fiber creates many problems. Too much of fiber intake may also be the reason behind your discomforts. You should keep a balance in fiber intake, after monitoring how much you take each day. You can get specific fiber addictive by consuming citrus foods, flaxseeds and legumes.

CHAPTER 7

HERBAL THERAPY FOR IBS

Herbal therapy refers to utilization of plants and plant products to get relief from diseases and health conditions. It has been proved that herbal therapy has been in practice since ancient Chinese civilizations.

There are few sets of ingredients or herbal therapies designed for IBS as well. Ancient remedies look at the pattern of symptoms and address it, rather than looking into diseases and its progress. The method of herbal treatments has been modified according to the present day conditions. Both the health conditions and availability of ingredients have changed over time.

The most commonly used herbs for irritable bowel syndrome include:

- Licorice
- Cardamom
- Rhubarb

- Barley
- Tangerine peel
- Barley

The products are easily available in markets. Make sure about the quality of the product and from where you buy it. To get the best possible benefits, the herbal products should be of the finest quality and in its purest form.

Even though if you are doubtful about the benefits of using these herbal products, we assure you that there is no harm in trying it yourself. There have been studies on herbal products for IBS and it shows improvement in patients by lessening the severity of symptoms.

Here goes a list of additional herbal supplements that you can take that has been proven in IBS patients.

Ginger

Ginger is a common health supplement to be consumed in order to get relief from IBS symptoms. You can use ginger in several ways. Extract the ginger juice and consume a few drops of it daily. It will help anti inflammatory conditions, improve the quality of gastric system and help intestines to perform their functions in a better way.

Peppermint Oil

Another common herbal ingredient in the treatment of gastrointestinal conditions is pepper oil. It has been proved that peppermint oil is good for IBS sufferers. But be careful when you consume too much of peppermint oil, as it may cause heartburn.

Peppermint oil helps in different ways. It decreases the amount of muscle spasm that your GI tract undergoes.

Moreover, it gives you relief from abdominal pain and bloating.

You can add few drops of peppermint oil to your drinks, which will help you in controlling the symptoms of IBS.

Artichoke Leaf Extract

Artichoke leaf extracts has been proven useful throughout Europe. It will help in improvement of the secretions of the bile. However, proper research and study on this topic is yet to start.

Others

There are more herbal products that you can take to get relief from constipation. To name a few of common products, rhubarb, senna, cascara, aloe etc are proven beneficial. You can consume a small amount daily as well as take in the form of supplemental pills.

IBS Diet (Irritable Bowel Syndrome)

CHAPTER 8

PROBIOTICS FOR IBS

Probiotics is another component that can be helpful for IBS sufferers. Probiotics are organisms that help to regulate the bacteria within the intestines. It is helpful for individuals with IBS, as it alters the intestinal flora. You will find relief from the symptoms of IBS by balancing these bacteria.

The bacterium, which lies inside the intestinal flora, helps to correct the function of GI tract. It also helps to keep your immune system intact and provide secretion of fluids.

Probiotics is used to stimulate the intestinal flora, as natural bacteria can help in treating IBS. Studies prove that probiotics have been beneficial in reducing the amount of abdominal pain in many individuals. The reduction of gas is also evident with the use of probiotics. In some people, it also helps in better functioning of the bowel.

You can purchase probiotics easily from health food stores as well as online and in your local area. It is an assumption that probiotics is really helpful in people with IBS, but scientific studies are still on the way.

CHAPTER 9

PREVENTION

IBS is not a condition which you need to be constantly worried about. You can think and be prepared to reduce the symptoms of IBS. Since we cannot point out the exact reason behind IBS in each person, it is important to know the symptoms and prevent it in whatever ways possible.

Prevention is best tool to fight against IBS. There are several things that you need to keep in mind when it comes to preventing the onset of irritable bowel syndrome symptoms.

Here goes some essential information on prevention of the symptoms related to IBS:

The Diet you follow

A proper diet has a major role to play in fixing the quality of your life. You can follow a proper diet in many ways. We recommend you to get through the eating diaries. Find out the food items that worsens the symptoms of IBS in you, and make sure you don't include those foods in your diet. Elimination diet is very helpful, but you should know that well balanced diet is also very important for good health.

You should also be careful about consuming the right amount of fiber foods. If you are suffering from constipation, it will be good to take additional source of fiber supplements.

Get Your Exercise

Exercise is an integral part of life to maintain proper health. Exercise can be or any sorts like yoga, walking for few minutes every day, aerobics etc. the best benefit of exercising regularly is that it decreases stress levels, which in turn controls symptoms of IBS.

Mind Therapy

Mind's health is also very important and that is why we suggest counseling. If you have a healthy mind, it will be helpful in reducing the symptoms of IBS. Meditation is a great tool to improve the health of mind. Give time to relax yourself and clear your mind, and in turn it will help you to reduce stress. You can take a relaxing bath after coming home or relax in bed for few moments before sleep, to get relief of daily stress.

Breathing

Practicing the right breathing technique also helps in fighting against IBS. You will probably breathing from your chest now, but you can learn to breathe from diaphragm by proper practice. It helps to reduce stress levels.

Are you confused about breathing exercise and its relation to IBS? During deep breathe in and breathe out, the stomach muscles expand. You will get relief from the extreme pain caused by IBS when the stomach muscles expand. In that way, you can reduce the pain and feel better.

As pointed out earlier, prevention is your goal when fighting IBS. Even if you can't manage to try out these prevention techniques, you can put aside twenty minutes every day to do something that is relaxing for you, be it anything. It will make you feel better and thus reduce the frequency of IBS symptoms.

If you practice one or two preventive measures, it will make a great difference in your well being and health..

IBS Diet (Irritable Bowel Syndrome)

CONCLUSION

Irritable bowel syndrome is a condition that may stay with you for longer period. You can lessen the frequency of symptoms and reduce it easily, provided you follow certain effective tools and methods to prevent it.

Your body reacts to every food you eat, be it good or bad. By determining the foods that make you suffer and limiting or removing them from diet, will result in your overall health. By eating a well-balanced diet and restricting foods that trigger your IBS symptoms, you can control the frequency of it.

Manage your diet. Determine the foods that worsen your symptoms. Get your fiber. Don't eat too much in one sitting. Relieve stress. Prevention is the best medicine. Use any of our recommended methods to manage stress effectively.

Eliminating IBS symptoms is not possible, and rather a challenge. The best thing you can do is to start with step one and work through all of them. Remember you should not try to implement a lot of change at once. Instead, work on improving your health, by one at a time. IBS can be conquered through it.

Thank you and good luck!

WaraWaran Roongruangsri

IBS Diet (Irritable Bowel Syndrome)